The Ultimate Intermittent Fasting 16/8 Guide

Discover How to Reset your Metabolism and Learn to Cook Healthy and Tasty Recipes. Quick and Easy Cookbook to Follow.

Carol Lamm

Additionally, the information in the following pages is intended only for informational purposes and should thus be thought of as universal. As befitting its nature, it is presented without assurance regarding its prolonged validity or interim quality. Trademarks that are mentioned are done without written consent and can in no way be considered an endorsement from the trademark holder.

Table of Contents

BREAKFAST

1. Turkey and Scrambled Eggs Breakfast

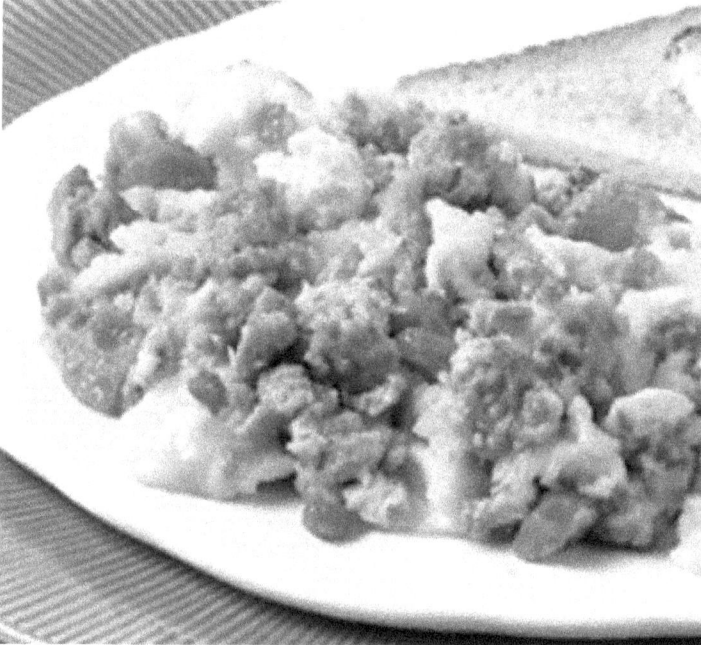

Preparation time: 10 minutes

Cooking time: 15 minutes

Servings: 2

Ingredients:

- 4 slices avocado
- Salt and pepper to taste
- 4 slices bacon, diced
- 4 turkey breast slices, cooked
- 4 tbsp. coconut oil
- 4 eggs, whisked

Directions:

1. Heat a pan over medium heat.
2. Add bacon slices and brown all over.
3. Heat oil in another pan.
4. Add eggs, salt, and pepper, and scramble.
5. Divide turkey breast slices, bacon, scrambled eggs, and avocado slices on 2 plates and serve.

Nutrition: Calories: 791 Fat: 64.3g Carb: 8.8g Protein: 41.8g

2. Breakfast Cereal

Preparation time: 5 minutes

Cooking time: 3 minutes

Servings: 2

Ingredients:

- ½ cup shredded coconut, unsweetened
- 4 tsp. butter
- 2 cups almond milk, unsweetened
- 1 tbsp. stevia
- Pinch of salt
- 2 tbsp. macadamia nuts, chopped
- 2 tbsp. walnuts, chopped
- 1/3 cup flaxseed

Directions:

1. Melt the butter in a pan.
2. Add the coconut, milk, salt, nuts, flaxseed, and stevia, and stir well.
3. Cook for 3 minutes and stir again.
4. Remove from heat. Set aside for 10 minutes.
5. Serve.

Nutrition: Calories: 588 Fat: 48g Carb: 6.8g Protein: 16.5g

3.   Best Intermittent Bread

Preparation time: 10 minutes

Cooking time: 30 minutes

Servings: 20

Ingredients:

- 1 ½ cup almond flour
- 6 drops liquid stevia
- 1 pinch Pink Himalayan salt
- ¼ tsp. cream of tartar
- 3 tsp. baking powder
- ¼ cup butter, melted
- 6 large eggs, separated

Directions:

1. Preheat the oven to 375F.
2. To the egg whites, add cream of tartar and beat until soft peaks are formed.
3. In a food processor, combine stevia, salt, baking powder, almond flour, melted butter, 1/3 of the beaten egg whites, and egg yolks. Mix well.
4. Then add the remaining 2/3 of the egg whites and gently process until fully mixed. Don't over mix.

5. Put a grease on a (8 x 4) loaf pan and pour the mixture in it.
6. Bake for 30 minutes.
7. Enjoy.

Nutrition: Calories: 90, Fat: 7g, Carb: 2g, Protein: 3g

4.   Bread De Soul

reparation time:10 minutes

Cooking time: 45 minutes

Servings: 16

Ingredients:

- ¼ tsp. cream of tartar
- 2 ½ tsp. baking powder
    - tsp. xanthan gum
- 1/3 tsp. baking soda
- ½ tsp. salt
- 2/3 cup unflavored whey protein
- ¼ cup olive oil
- ¼ cup heavy whipping cream
- drops of sweet leaf stevia
- eggs
- ¼ cup butter
- 12 oz. softened cream cheese

Directions:

1. Preheat the oven to 325F.
2. In a bowl, microwave cream cheese and butter for 1 minute.

3. Remove and blend well with a hand mixer.
4. Add olive oil, eggs, heavy cream, and few drops of sweetener and blend well.
5. Put together the dry ingredients in a separate bowl.
6. Combine the dry ingredients with the wet ingredients and mix with a spoon. Don't use a hand blender to avoid whipping it too much.
7. Grease a bread pan and pour the mixture into the pan.
8. Bake in the oven until golden brown for about 45 minutes.
9. Cool and serve.

Nutrition: Calories: 200, Fat: 15.2g, Carb: 1.8g, Protein: 10g

5. Chia Seed Bread

Preparation time: 10 minutes

Cooking time: 4 minutes

Servings: 16

Ingredients:

- ½ tsp. xanthan gum
- ½ cup butter
- 2 Tbsp. coconut oil
- Tbsp. baking powder
- Tbsp. sesame seeds
- Tbsp. chia seeds
- ½ tsp. salt
- ¼ cup sunflower seeds
- 2 cups almond flour
- 7 eggs

Directions:

1. Preheat the oven to 350F.
2. Beat eggs in a bowl for 1 to 2 minutes.
3. Beat in the xanthan gum and combine coconut oil and melted butter into eggs, beating continuously.

4. Set aside the sesame seeds, but add the rest of the ingredients.
5. Get a loaf pan with baking paper and place the mixture in it. Top the mixture with sesame seeds.
6. Bake in the oven for about 35 to 40 minutes.

Nutrition: Calories: 405, Fat: 37g, Carb: 4g, Protein: 14g

6. Special Intermittent Bread

Preparation time: 15 minutes

Cooking time: 40 minutes

Servings: 14

Ingredients:

- 2 tsp. baking powder
- ½ cup water
- 1Tbsp. poppy seeds
- 3cups fine ground almond meal
- 5 large eggs
- ½ cup olive oil
- ½ tsp. fine Himalayan salt

Directions:

1. Preheat oven to 400F.
2. In a bowl, combine salt, almond meal, and baking powder.
3. Drip in oil while mixing, until it forms a crumbly dough.
4. Make a little round hole in the middle of the dough and pour eggs into the middle of the dough.

5. Pour water and whisk eggs together with the mixer in the small circle until it is frothy.

6. Start making larger circles to combine the almond meal mixture with the dough until you have a smooth and thick batter.

7. Line your loaf pan with parchment paper.

8. Pour batter into the loaf pan and sprinkle poppy seeds on top.

9. Bake in the oven for 40 minutes in the center rack until firm and golden brown.

10.   Cool in the oven for 30 minutes.

11.   Slice and serve.

Nutrition: Calories: 227, Fat: 21g, Carb: 4g, Protein: 7g

7.   Intermittent Fluffy Cloud Bread

Preparation time: 25 minutes

Cooking time: 25 minutes

Servings: 3

Ingredients:

- pinch salt
- ½ Tbsp. ground psyllium husk powder
- ½ Tbsp. baking powder
- ¼ tsp. cream of tarter
- eggs, separated
- ½ cup, cream cheese

Directions:

1. Preheat oven to 300F.
2. Whisk egg whites in a bowl until soft peaks are formed.
3. Mix egg yolks with cream cheese, salt, cream of tartar, psyllium husk powder, and baking powder in a bowl.
4. Fold in the egg whites carefully and transfer to the baking tray.
5. Place in the oven and bake for 25 minutes.

6. Remove from the oven and serve.

Nutrition: Calories: 185, Fat: 16.4g, Carb: 3.9g, Protein: 6.6

8.   Splendid Low-Carb Bread

Preparation time: 15 minutes

Cooking time: 60 to 70 minutes

Servings: 12

Ingredients:

- ½ tsp. herbs, such as basil, rosemary, or oregano
- ½ tsp. garlic or onion powder
- Tbsp. baking powder
- 5 Tbsp. psyllium husk powder
- ½ cup almond flour
- ½ cup coconut flour
- ¼ tsp. salt
- ½ cup egg whites
- Tbsp. oil or melted butter
- Tbsp. apple cider vinegar
- 1/3 to ¾ cup hot water

Directions:

1. Put a grease on a loaf pan and preheat the oven to 350F.

2. In a bowl, whisk the salt, psyllium husk powder, onion or garlic powder, coconut flour, almond flour, and baking powder.
3. Stir in egg whites, oil, and apple cider vinegar. Bit by bit add the hot water, stirring until dough increase in size. Do not add too much water.
4. Mold the dough into a rectangle and transfer to grease loaf pan.
5. Bake in the oven for 60 to 70 minutes, or until crust feels firm and brown on top.
6. Cool and serve.

Nutrition: Calories: 97, Fat: 5.7g, Carb: 7.5g, Protein: 4.1g

9. Coconut Flour Almond Bread

Preparation time: 10 minutes

Cooking time: 30 minutes

Servings: 4

Ingredients:

- Tbsp. butter, melted
- 1Tbsp. coconut oil, melted
- 6 eggs
- 1 tsp. baking soda
- Tbsp. ground flaxseed
- 1 ½ Tbsp. psyllium husk powder
- 5 Tbsp. coconut flour
- 1 ½ cup almond flour

Directions:

1. Preheat the oven to 400F.
2. Mix the eggs in a bowl for a few minutes.
3. Add in the butter and coconut oil and mix once more for 1 minute.
4. Add the almond flour, coconut flour, baking soda, psyllium husk, and ground flaxseed to the mixture. Let sit for 15 minutes.

5. Grease the loaf pan with coconut oil. Pour the mixture in the pan.
6. Put in the oven. Bake until a toothpick in it comes out dry, about 25 minutes.

Nutrition: Calories: 475, Fat: 38g, Carb: 7g, Protein: 19g

LUNCH

10. Cheesy Chicken Cauliflower

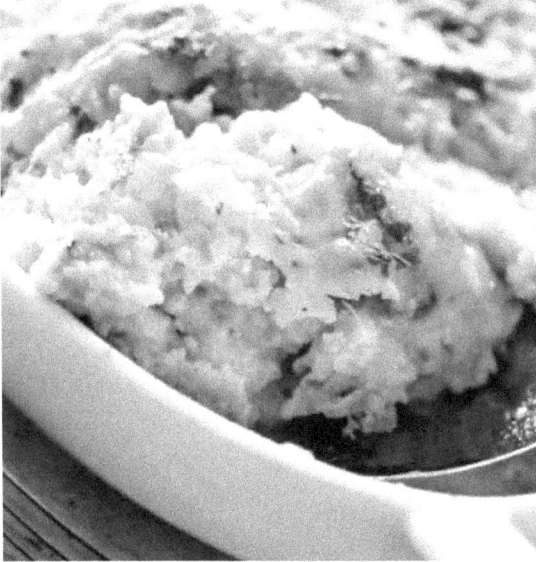

Preparation Time: 5 minutes

Cooking Time: 10 minutes

Servings: 4

Ingredients:

- 2 cups cauliflower florets, chopped
- ½ cup red bell pepper, chopped

- 1 cup roasted chicken, shredded (Lunch Recipes: Roasted Lemon Chicken Sandwich)
- ¼ cup shredded cheddar cheese
- 1 tablespoon. butter
- 1 tablespoon. sour cream
- Salt and pepper to taste

Directions:

1. Stir fry the cauliflower and peppers in the butter over medium heat until the veggies are tender.
2. Add the chicken and cook until the chicken is warmed through.
3. Add the remaining ingredients and stir until the cheese is melted.
4. Serve warm.

Nutrition: Calories: 144 kcal Carbs: 4 g Fat: 8.5 g Protein: 13.2 g.

11. Chicken Avocado Salad

Preparation Time: 7 minutes

Cooking Time: 10 minutes

Servings: 4

Ingredients:

- 1 cup roasted chicken, shredded (Lunch Recipes: Roasted Lemon Chicken Sandwich)
- 1 bacon strip, cooked and chopped
- 1/2 medium avocado, chopped
- ¼ cup cheddar cheese, grated
- 1 hard-boiled egg, chopped
- 1 cup romaine lettuce, chopped
- 1 tablespoon. olive oil
- 1 tablespoon. apple cider vinegar
- Salt and pepper to taste

Directions:

1. Create the dressing by mixing apple cider vinegar, oil, salt and pepper.
2. Combine all the other ingredients in a mixing bowl.
3. Drizzle with the dressing and toss.

4. Can be refrigerated for up to 3 days.

Nutrition: Calories: 220 kcal Carbs: 2.8 g Fat: 16.7 g Protein: 14.8 g.

12. Chicken Broccoli Dinner

Preparation Time: 10 minutes

Cooking Time: 5 minutes

Servings: 1

Ingredients:

- 1 roasted chicken leg (Lunch Recipes: Roasted Lemon Chicken Sandwich)
- ½ cup broccoli florets
- ½ tablespoon. unsalted butter, softened
- 2 garlic cloves, minced
- Salt and pepper to taste

Directions:

1. Boil the broccoli in lightly salted water for 5 minutes. Drain the water from the pot and keep the broccoli in the pot. Keep the lid on to keep the broccoli warm.
2. Mix all the butter, garlic, salt and pepper in a small bowl to create garlic butter.
3. Place the chicken, broccoli and garlic butter.

Nutrition: Calories: 257 kcal Carbs: 5.1 g Fat: 14 g Protein: 27.4 g.

13. Easy Meatballs

Preparation Time: 10 minutes

Cooking Time: 20 minutes

Servings: 4

Ingredients:

- 1 lb. ground beef
- 1 egg, beaten
- Salt and pepper to taste
- 1 teaspoon garlic powder
- 1 teaspoon onion powder
- 2 tablespoons. butter
- ¼ cup mayonnaise
- ¼ cup pickled jalapeños
- 1 cup cheddar cheese, grated

Directions

1. Combine the cheese, mayonnaise, pickled jalapenos, salt, pepper, garlic powder and onion powder in a large mixing bowl.
2. Add the beef and egg and combine using clean hands.
3. Form large meatballs. Makes about 12.

4. Fry the meatballs in the butter over medium heat for about 4 minutes on each side or until golden brown.

5. Serve warm with an intermittent-friendly side.

6. The meatball mixture can also be used to make a meatloaf. Just preheat your oven to 400 degrees F, press the mixture into a loaf pan and bake for about 30 minutes or until the top is golden brown.

7. Can be refrigerated for up to 5 days or frozen for up to 3 months.

Nutrition: Calories: 454 kcal Carbs: 5 g Fat: 28.2 g Protein: 43.2 g.

14. Chicken Casserole

Preparation Time: 10 minutes

Cooking Time: 40 minutes

Servings: 8

Ingredients:

- 1 lb. boneless chicken breasts, cut into 1" cubes
- 2 tablespoons. butter
- 4 tablespoons. green pesto
- 1 cup heavy whipping cream
- ¼ cup green bell peppers, diced
- 1 cup feta cheese, diced
- 1 garlic clove, minced
- Salt and pepper to taste

Directions

1. Preheat your oven to 400 degrees F.
2. Season the chicken with salt and pepper then batch fry in the butter until golden brown.
3. Place the fried chicken pieces in a baking dish. Add the feta cheese, garlic and bell peppers.

4. Combine the pesto and heavy cream in a bowl. Pour on top of the chicken mixture and spread with a spatula.
5. Bake for 30 minutes or until the casserole is light brown around the edges.
6. Serve warm.
7. Can be refrigerated for up to 5 days and frozen for 2 weeks.

Nutrition: Calories: 294 kcal Carbs: 1.7 g Fat: 22.7 g Protein: 20.1 g.

15. Lemon Baked Salmon

Preparation Time: 10 minutes

Cooking Time: 30 minutes

Servings: 4

Ingredients:

- 1 lb. salmon
- 1 tablespoon. olive oil
- Salt and pepper to taste
- 1 tablespoon. butter
- 1 lemon, thinly sliced
- 1 tablespoon. lemon juice

Directions:

1. Preheat your oven to 400 degrees F.
2. Grease a baking dish with the olive oil and place the salmon skin-side down.
3. Season the salmon with salt and pepper then top with the lemon slices.
4. Slice half the butter and place over the salmon.
5. Bake for 20minutes or until the salmon flakes easily.

6. Melt the remaining butter in a saucepan. When it starts to bubble, remove from heat and allow to cool before adding the lemon juice.
7. Drizzle the lemon butter over the salmon and Serve warm.

Nutrition: Calories: 211 kcal Carbs: 1.5 g Fat: 13.5 g Protein: 22.2 g.

16. Cauliflower Mash

Preparation Time: 10 minutes

Cooking Time: 5 minutes

Servings: 8

Ingredients:

- 4 cups cauliflower florets, chopped
- 1 cup grated parmesan cheese
- 6 tablespoons. butter
- ½ lemon, juice and zest
- Salt and pepper to taste

Directions:

1. Boil the cauliflower in lightly salted water over high heat for 5 minutes or until the florets are tender but still firm.
2. Strain the cauliflower in a colander and add the cauliflower to a food processor
3. Add the remaining ingredients and pulse the mixture to a smooth and creamy consistency
4. Serve with protein like salmon, chicken or meatballs.
5. Can be refrigerated for up to 3 days.

Nutrition: Calories: 101 kcal Carbs: 3.1 g Fat: 9.5 g Protein: 2.2 g.

17. Roasted Chicken Soup

Preparation Time: 10 minutes

Cooking Time: 25 minutes

Servings: 6

Ingredients:

- 4 cups roasted chicken, shredded (Lunch Recipes: Roasted Lemon Chicken Sandwich)
- 2 tablespoons. butter
- 2 celery stalks, chopped
- 1 cup mushrooms, sliced
- 4 cups green cabbage, sliced into strips
- 2 garlic cloves, minced
- 6 cups chicken broth
- 1 carrot, sliced
- Salt and pepper to taste
- 1 tablespoon. garlic powder
- 1 tablespoon. onion powder

Directions:

1. Sauté the celery, mushrooms and garlic in the butter in a pot over medium heat for 4 minutes.

2. Add broth, carrots, garlic powder, onion powder, salt, and pepper.

3. Simmer for 10 minutes or until the vegetables are tender.

4. Add the chicken and cabbage and simmer for another 10 minutes or until the cabbage is tender.

5. Serve warm.

6. Can be refrigerated for up to 3 days or frozen for up to 1 month.

Nutrition: Calories: 279 kcal Carbs: 7.5 g Fat: 12.3 g Protein: 33.4 g.

DINNER

18. Clean Salmon with Soy Sauce

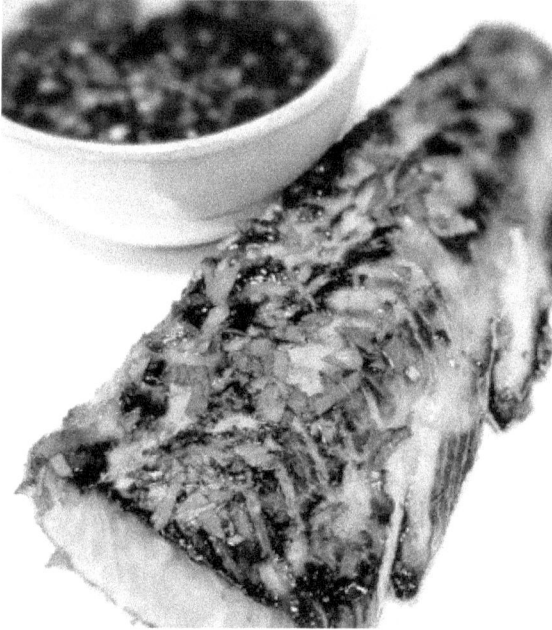

Preparation Time: 10 minutes

Cooking Time: 30 minutes

Servings: 2

Ingredients:

- 2 Salmon fillets
- 2 tbsp Avocado oil

- 2 tbsp Soy sauce
- 1 tbsp Garlic powder
- 2 tbsp fresh Dill to garnish
- Salt and Pepper, to taste

Directions:

1. To make the marinade, thoroughly mix the soy sauce, avocado oil, salt, pepper and garlic powder into a bowl. Dip salmon in the mixture and place in the refrigerator for 20 minutes.
2. Transfer the contents to the Instant pot. Seal, set on Manual and cook for 10 minutes on high pressure.
3. When ready, do a quick release. Serve topped with the fresh dill.

Nutrition: Calories 512, Protein 65g, Net Carbs 3.2g, Fat 21g

19. Simple Salmon with Eggs

Preparation Time: 2 minutes

Cooking Time: 5 minutes

Servings: 3

Ingredients:

- 1 lb. Salmon, cooked, mashed
- 2 Eggs, whisked
- 2 Onions, chopped
- 2 stalks celery, chopped
- 1 cup Parsley, chopped
- 2 tbsp Olive oil
- Salt and Pepper, to taste

Directions:

1. Mix salmon, onion, celery, parsley, and salt and pepper, in a bowl. Form into 6 patties about 1 inch thick and dip them in the whisked eggs. Heat oil in the Instant pot on Sauté mode.
2. Add the patties to the pot and cook on both sides, for about 5 minutes and transfer to the plate. Allow to cool and serve.

Nutrition: Calories 331, Protein 38g, Net Carbs 5.3g, Fat 16g

20. Easy Shrimp

Preparation Time: 4 minutes

Cooking Time: 5 minutes

Servings: 2

Ingredients:

- 1 lb. Shrimp, peeled and deveined
- 1 Garlic cloves, crushed
- 1 tbsp Butter.
- A pinch of red Pepper
- Salt and Pepper, to taste
- 1 cup Parsley, chopped

Directions:

1. Melt butter on Sauté mode. Add shrimp, garlic, red pepper, salt and pepper.
2. Cook for 5 minutes, stirring occasionally the shrimp until pink. Serve topped with parsley.

Nutrition: Calories 245, Protein 45g, Net Carbs 4.8g, Fat 4g

21. Scallops with Mushroom Special

Preparation Time: 15 minutes

Cooking Time: 20 minutes

Servings: 2

Ingredients:

- 1 lb. Scallops
- 2 Onions, chopped
- 1 tbsp Butter
- 2 tbsp Olive oil
- 1 cup Mushrooms
- Salt and Pepper, to taste
- 1 tbsp Lemon juice
- ½ cup Whipping Cream
- 1 tbsp chopped fresh Parsley

Directions:

1. Heat the oil on Sauté. Add onions, butter, mushrooms, salt and pepper. Cook for 3 to 5 minutes. Add the lemon juice and scallops. Lock the lid and set to Manual mode.
2. Cook for 15 minutes on High pressure.

3. When ready, do a quick pressure release and carefully open the lid. Top with a drizzle of cream and fresh parsley.

Nutrition: Calories 312, Protein 31g, Net Carbs 7.3g, Fat 10.4g

22. Delicious Creamy Crab Meat

Preparation Time: 5 minutes

Cooking Time: 10 minutes

Servings: 3

Ingredients:

- 1 lb. Crab meat
- ½ cup Cream cheese
- 2 tbsp Mayonnaise
- Salt and Pepper, to taste
- 1 tbsp Lemon juice
- 1 cup Cheddar cheese, shredded

Directions:

1. Mix mayo, cream cheese, salt and pepper, and lemon juice in a bowl. Add in crab meat and make small balls. Place the balls inside the pot. Seal the lid and press Manual.
2. Cook for 10 minutes on High pressure. When done, allow the pressure to release naturally for 10 minutes. Sprinkle the cheese over and serve!

Nutrition: Calories 443, Protein 41g, Net Carbs 2.5g, Fat 30.4g

23. Creamy Broccoli Stew

Preparation Time: 10 minutes

Cooking Time: 20 minutes

Servings: 4

Ingredients:

- 1 cup Heavy Cream
- 3 oz. Parmesan cheese
- 1 cup Broccoli florets
- 2 Carrots, sliced
- ½ tbsp Garlic paste
- ¼ tbsp Turmeric powder
- Salt and black Pepper, to taste
- ½ cup Vegetable broth
- 2 tbsp Butter

Directions:

1. Melt butter on Sauté mode. Add garlic and sauté for 30 seconds. Add broccoli and carrots, and cook until soft, for 2-3 minutes. Season with salt and pepper.
2. Stir in the vegetable broth and seal the lid. Cook on Meat/Stew mode for 40 minutes. When ready,

do a quick pressure release. Stir in the heavy cream.

Nutrition: Calories 239, Protein 8g, Net Carbs 5.1g, Fat 21.4g

24. No Crust Tomato and Spinach Quiche

Preparation Time: 10 minutes

Cooking Time: 30 minutes

Servings: 3

Ingredients:

- 14 large Eggs
- 1 cup Full Milk
- Salt to taste
- Ground Black Pepper to taste
- 4 cups fresh Baby Spinach, chopped
- 2 Tomatoes, diced
- 3 Scallions, sliced
- 1 Tomato, sliced into firm rings
- ½ cup Parmesan Cheese, shredded
- Water for boiling

Directions:

1. Place the trivet in the pot and pour in 1 ½ cups of water. Break the eggs into a bowl, add salt, pepper, and milk and whisk it. Share the diced tomatoes, spinach and scallions into 3 ramekins,

gently stir, and arrange 3 slices of tomatoes on top in each ramekin.

2. Sprinkle with Parmesan cheese. Gently place the ramekins in the pot, and seal the lid. Select Manual and cook on High Pressure for 20 minutes. Once ready, quickly release the pressure.

3. Carefully remove the ramekins and use a paper towel to tap soak any water from the steam that sits on the quiche. Brown the top of the quiche with a fire torch.

Nutrition: Calories 310, Protein 12g, Net Carbs 0g, Fat 27g

25. Peas Soup

Preparation time: 10 minutes

Cooking time: 10 minutes

Servings: 4

Ingredients:

- 1 white onion, chopped
- 1 tablespoon olive oil
- 1 quart veggie stock
- 2 eggs
- 3 tablespoons lemon juice
- 2 cups peas
- 2 tablespoons parmesan, grated
- Salt and black pepper to the taste

Directions:

1. Heat up a pot with the oil over medium-high heat, add the onion and sauté for 4 minutes.
2. Add the rest of the ingredients except the eggs, bring to a simmer and cook for 4 minutes.
3. Add whisked eggs, stir the soup, cook for 2 minutes more, divide into bowls and serve.

Nutrition: Calories 293, fat 11.2 fiber 3.4, carbs 27, protein 4.45

SNACKS

26. Intermittent Seed Crispy Crackers

Preparation Time: 60 minutes

Cooking Time: 55 minutes

Servings: 30

Ingredients:

- 1/3 cup almond flour
- 1/3 cup sunflower seed kernels
- 1/3 cup pumpkin seed kernels
- 1/3 cup flaxseed
- 1/3 cup chia seeds
- 1 tbsp ground psyllium husk powder
- 1 tsp salt
- ¼ cup melted coconut oil
- 1 cup boiling water

Directions:

1. Preheat the oven to 300 degrees.

2. Stir all dry ingredients together in a medium-sized bowl until thoroughly mixed.
3. Add coconut oil and boiling water to dry ingredients and stir until all ingredients are mixed well.
4. On a flat surface, roll the dough between two pieces of parchment paper until approximately ⅛ inch thick.
5. Slide the dough, still between parchment paper onto a baking sheet.
6. Remove the top layer of parchment paper and place dough on a baking sheet into the oven.
7. Bake 40 minutes until golden brown.
8. Score the top of the dough into cracker sized pieces.
9. Leave in the oven to cool down.
10. When the big cracker is cool, break into pieces.
11. These crackers can be stored in an airtight container after they are completely cool.

Nutrition: Calories: 61 Carbohydrates: 1g Protein: .2g Fat: .6g Sodium: 90 mg

27. Parmesan Crackers

Preparation time: 10 minutes

Cooking time: 5 minutes

Servings: 8

Ingredients:

- Butter – 1 tsp.
- Full-fat parmesan – 8 ounces, shredded

Directions:

1. Preheat the oven to 400F.
2. Line a baking sheet with parchment paper and lightly grease the paper with the butter.
3. Spoon the parmesan cheese onto the baking sheet in mounds, spread evenly apart.
4. Spread out the mounds with the back of a spoon until they are flat.
5. Bake about 5 minutes, or until the center are still pale, and edges are browned.
6. Remove, cool, and serve.

Nutrition: Calories: 133 Fat: 11g Carb: 1g Protein: 11g Sodium: 483 mg

28. Deviled Eggs

Preparation time: 15 minutes

Cooking time: 10 minutes

Servings: 12

Ingredients:

- Large eggs – 6, hardboiled, peeled, and halved lengthwise
- Creamy mayonnaise – ¼ cup
- Avocado – ¼, chopped
- Swiss cheese – ¼ cup, shredded
- Dijon mustard – ½ tsp.
- Ground black pepper
- Bacon slices – 6, cooked and chopped

Directions

1. Remove the yolks and place them in a bowl. Place the whites on a plate, hollow-side up.
2. Mash the yolks with a fork and add Dijon mustard, cheese, avocado, and mayonnaise. Mix well and season yolk mixture with the black pepper.

3. Spoon the yolk mixture back into the egg white hollows and top each egg half with the chopped bacon.
4. Serve.

Nutrition: Calories: 85 Fat: 7g Carb: 2g Protein: 6g Sodium: 108 mg

29. Almond Garlic Crackers

Preparation time: 10 minutes

Cooking time: 15 minutes

Servings: 4

Ingredients:

- Almond flour – ½ cup
- Ground flaxseed – ½ cup
- Shredded Parmesan cheese – 1/3 cup
- Garlic powder – 1 tsp.
- Salt – ½ tsp.
- Water as needed

Directions:

1. Line a baking sheet with parchment paper and preheat the oven to 400F.
2. In a bowl, mix salt, Parmesan cheese, garlic powder, water, ground flaxseed, and almond meal. Set aside for 3 to 5 minutes.
3. Put dough on the baking sheet and cover with plastic wrap. Flatten the dough with a rolling pin.
4. Remove the plastic wrap and score the dough with a knife to make dents.

5. Bake in the oven for 15 minutes.

6. Remove, cool, and break into individual crackers.

Nutrition: Calories: 96 Fat: 14g Carb: 4g Protein: 4g Sodium: 446 mg

30. Bacon Ranch Fat Bombs

Preparation time: 15 minutes

Cooking time: 15 minutes

Servings:4

Ingredients:

- 8 oz full-fat cream cheese, softened
- 1 tbsp ranch dressing dry mix
- 2 slices bacon

Directions:

1. Preheat the oven to 375°F.
2. Cook the bacon strips on a baking tray for 15 minutes. Let cool, then crumble.
3. In a bowl, add cream cheese and sprinkle with ranch dressing dry mix. Stir in the bacon. Mix thoroughly.
4. Form a ball out of 1 tbsp of the mixture. Repeat to form 3 more bombs. Refrigerate for 2 hours. Serve.

Nutrition: Total Carbs – 9.5 g Net Carbs – 2.7 g Fat – 38.9 g Protein – 11.4 g Calories – 419

31. Salmon Mascarpone Balls

Preparation time: 7 minutes

Cooking time: 0

Servings: 6

Ingredients:

- 3 oz smoked salmon, chopped
- 3 oz mascarpone
- ½ tsp maple flavor
- ½ tsp chives, chopped
- 3 Tbsp hemp hearts

Directions:

1. In a small food processor, combine salmon, mascarpone, maple flavor, and chives. Pulse a few times until blended together.
2. Form mixture into 6 balls.
3. Put hemp hearts on a medium plate and roll individual balls through to coat evenly.
4. Serve immediately or refrigerate up to 3 days.

Nutrition: Total Carbs – 1 g Net Carbs – 0 g Fat – 5 g Protein – 3 g Calories – 65

32. Bacon, Artichoke & Onion Fat Bombs

Preparation time: 15 minutes

Cooking time: 8 minutes

Servings: 4

Ingredients:

- 2 bacon slices
- 2 tbsp ghee
- ½ large onion, peeled, diced
- 1 garlic clove, minced
- ⅓ cup canned artichoke hearts, sliced
- ¼ cup sour cream
- ¼ cup mayonnaise
- 1 tbsp lemon juice
- ¼ cup Swiss cheese, grated
- Salt, pepper to taste
- 4 avocado halves, pitted

Directions:

1. In a hot skillet, fry the bacon for 5 minutes. Let cool, then crumble.

2. Cook the onion and garlic using ghee for 3 minutes.
3. Combine the onion and garlic with the bacon and the remaining ingredients. Mix well. Season with salt and pepper. Refrigerate 30 minutes. Fill the avocado halves with the mixture and serve.

Nutrition: Total Carbs – 10 g Net Carbs – 4 g Fat – 39.6 g Protein – 6.6 g Calories – 408

33. Spicy Bacon and Avocado Balls

Preparation time: 45 minutes

Cooking time: 8 minutes

Servings: 6

Ingredients:

- 4 slices bacon
- 1 medium avocado
- 2 Tbsp coconut oil
- 1 Tbsp bacon fat
- 1 Tbsp green onions, finely chopped
- 2 Tbsp cilantro, finely chopped
- 1 small jalapeño pepper, seeded, finely chopped
- ¼ tsp sea salt

Directions:

1. Over medium heat, cook bacon until golden, about 4 minutes each side.
2. Drain bacon on a paper towel. Save bacon fat for later.
3. Once bacon is cool, chop 2 slices into crumbles.
4. Cut remaining 2 slices into 3 pieces each.
5. Smash avocado with a fork in a small bowl.

6. Add coconut oil and cooled bacon fat to avocado.

7. Add onion, cilantro, jalapeño, salt, and bacon crumbles. Blend well.

8. Refrigerate for 30 minutes.

9. Form mixture into 6 balls.

10. Place remaining 6 bacon pieces on a plate, then top each with an avocado ball.

11. Serve or refrigerate up to 3 days.

Nutrition: Total Carbs – 3 g Net Carbs – 1 g Fat – 18 g Protein – 3 g Calories – 181

MEATS

34. Beef Mini Meatloaves With Bacon Wrappings

Preparation time: 10 minutes

Cooking time: 30 minutes

Servings: 8

Ingredients:

- 1pound (454 g) ground beef
- ⅓ cup nutritional yeast
- ¾ teaspoon ground gray sea salt
- ¼ cup low-carb tomato sauce
- 1 tablespoon prepared yellow mustard
- ¼ teaspoon ground black pepper
- 8 (1-ounce / 28-g) strips bacon

Directions:

1. Preheat the oven to 350°F (180°C).

2. In a bowl, add the beef, yeast, salt, tomato sauce, mustard, and pepper. Mix well with your hands.

3. Make the mini meatloaves: Scoop out 1 tablespoon portions and roll to form a cylinder. Repeat with the remaining mixture to make 8 cylinders. Wrap each of the cylinders with one strip of bacon. Transfer the wrapped cylinders to a cast-iron pan (loose ends of the bacon facing down) with a spacing of ½ inch (1.25 cm) between cylinders.

4. Bake in the preheated oven for about 30 minutes or until an instant-read thermometer inserted in the center registers 165°F (74°C).

5. Adjust the oven broiler to high. Allow the mini meatloaves to broil for 2 minutes until the bacon is crispy.

6. Transfer to a serving platter to cool before serving.

Nutrition: calories: 295 fat: 21.2g total carbs: 3.2g fiber: 1.0g protein: 21.9g

35. Sloppy Joes

Preparation time: 15 minutes

Cooking time: 40 minutes

Servings: 8

Ingredients:

- ¼ cup plus 1½ teaspoons refined avocado oil
- 1 teaspoon cumin seeds
- 2 small minced cloves garlic
- 1 minced piece fresh ginger root
- ¼ cup red onions, finely diced
- 1 pound (454 g) ground beef
- 1⅔ cups low-carb tomato sauce
- 2 crushed whole dried chilis
- ¾ cup water
- 2 teaspoons curry powder
- ½ teaspoon paprika
- 1 teaspoon finely ground gray sea salt
- ⅓ cup raw macadamia nut halves
- 1 tablespoon apple cider vinegar
- ½ cup unsweetened coconut milk
- ¼ cup chopped fresh cilantro leaves, plus more for garnish

- 4 endives, leaves separated, plus more for garnish

Directions:

1. Make Sloppy Joes: Add ¼ cup oil, cumin seeds, garlic, ginger, and onions in a saucepan. Cook over medium heat for about 3 minutes until the onions are fragrant.
2. Add the beef to cook for about 8 minutes until it loses the pink color. Stir occasionally to break the beef into small clumps.
3. Add the tomato sauce, crushed chilis, water, curry powder, paprika, and salt and stir thoroughly to mix. Cover the lid partially to allow the steam to escape. Bring to a boil before adjusting the heat to medium-low to simmer for 25 minutes.
4. In a frying pan over medium-low heat, add the remaining oil and macadamia nuts. Roast for about 3 minutes until lightly golden. Toss constantly.
5. After 25 minutes of simmering, add the vinegar and coconut milk to the meat mixture. Adjust to medium-high heat and cook for about 5 minutes until thickened.

6. Add the cilantro and roasted nuts into the meat mixture. Stir well to mix.
7. Divide the endive leaves equally on 8 plates. Top with Sloppy Joes using a spoon.
8. Garnish the meal with extra cilantro and endives before serving.

Nutrition: calories: 340 | fat: 26.8g | total carbs: 8.1g | fiber: 2.7g | protein: 16.5g

36. Cheese, Olives and Sausage Casserole

Preparation time: 10 minutes

Cooking time: 15 minutes

Servings: 2

Ingredients:

- 3 oz sausage
- 1.5 oz green olives, sliced
- 2 eggs
- 4 oz coconut milk, unsweetened
- 3 tbsp grated cheddar cheese
- Seasoning:
- ¼ tsp ground black pepper
- 1/3 tsp salt
- 1/3 tsp mustard powder

Directions:

1. Take a medium skillet pan, place it over medium heat and when hot, add sausage, crumble it and cook for 5 minutes until cooked.

2. Meanwhile, crack eggs in a medium bowl, add milk, salt, black pepper, and mustard and whisk until blended.
3. When sausage had cooked, add sausage mixture into the eggs, add onion and olives, 2 tbsp cheese, and then stir until mixed.
4. Then spoon the mixture into a casserole dish, cover with a lid and let it refrigerate for 1 hour until chilled.
5. When ready to bake, Turn on the oven, then set it to 350 degrees F and let it preheat.
6. Sprinkle cheese on the top casserole and then bake it for 10 minutes until cheese has melted.
7. Serve.

Nutrition: 351 Calories; 30.6 g Fats; 15.7 g Protein; 1.7 g Net Carb; 0.9 g Fiber;

37. Curried Ground Sausage

Preparation time: 5 minutes

Cooking time: 15 minutes

Ingredients:

- 5 oz sausage, crumbled
- 1 green onion, sliced
- 2 oz spinach
- 1-ounce chicken bone broth
- 1-ounce whipping cream
- 1 tbsp avocado oil
- ½ tsp garlic powder
- 1 tbsp curry powder
- ¼ cup of water

Directions:

1. Take a medium saucepan, place it over medium heat, add ½ tbsp oil and when hot, add ground sausage and cook for 4 to 5 minutes until cooked.
2. When done, transfer sausage to a bowl, add remaining oil and when hot, add green onion, sprinkle with garlic powder and cook for 2 minutes until sauté.

3. Sprinkle with curry powder, continue cooking for 30 seconds until fragrant, pour in chicken broth and water, add sausage and spinach, stir until mixed and simmer for 5 minutes until thickened slightly.
4. Taste to adjust seasoning, stir in cream and then remove the pan from heat.
5. Serve.

Nutrition: 435 Calories; 42 g Fats; 12 g Protein; 1.4 g Net Carb; 0.8 g Fiber;

38. Portobello Mushrooms with Sausage and Cheese

Preparation time: 10 minutes

Cooking time: 20 minutes

Servings: 2

Ingredients:

- 2 Portobello mushroom caps
- 2 oz sausage
- 1 tbsp melted butter, unsalted
- 2 tbsp grated parmesan cheese
- 1/8 tsp garlic powder
- 1/8 tsp red chili powder
- ¼ tsp salt
- 2 tsp avocado oil

Directions:

1. Turn on the oven, then set it to 425 degrees F and let it preheat.
2. Meanwhile, remove the stems from mushroom caps, chop them and then brush the caps with butter inside-out.

3. Take a frying pan, place it over medium heat, add oil and when hot, add sausage, crumble it, sprinkle with garlic powder and then cook for 5 minutes until cooked.
4. Stir in mushroom stems, season with salt and black pepper, continue cooking for 3 minutes until cooked and then remove the pan from heat.
5. Distribute sausage-mushroom mixture into mushroom caps, sprinkle cheese, and red chili powder on top and then bake for 10 t0 12 minutes until mushroom caps have turned tender and cooked. Serve.

Nutrition: 310 Calories; 26 g Fats; 10.7 g Protein; 6.6 g Net Carb; 1.1 g Fiber;

39. Sausage and Cauliflower Rice

Preparation time: 5 minutes

Cooking time: 15 minutes;

Servings: 2

Ingredients:

- 7 oz grated cauliflower
- 3 oz sausage
- 1 green onion, sliced
- ½ tsp garlic powder
- 2 tbsp avocado oil
- 1/3 tsp salt
- ¼ tsp ground black pepper
- 6 tbsp water

Directions:

1. Take a medium skillet pan, place it over medium heat, add 1 tbsp oil and when hot, add sausage and cook for 4 to 5 minutes until nicely browned.
2. Switch heat to medium-low level, pour in 4 tbsp water and then simmer for 5 to 7 minutes until sausage has thoroughly cooked.

3. Transfer sausage to a bowl, wipe clean the pan, then return it over medium heat, add oil and when hot, add cauliflower rice and green onion, sprinkle with garlic powder, salt, and black pepper.
4. Stir until mixed, drizzle with 2 tbsp water, and cook for 5 minutes until softened.
5. Add sausage, stir until mixed, cook for 1 minute until hot and then serve.

Nutrition: 333 Calories; 31.3 g Fats; 9.1 g Protein; 0.8 g Net Carb; 2.5 g Fiber;

40. Cheesy Sausage and Egg Bake

Preparation time: 5 minutes

Cooking time: 18 minutes

Servings: 2

Ingredients:

- 4 oz sausage
- 1 egg
- 2 tbsp grated cheddar cheese
- 1 ½ tbsp grated mozzarella cheese
- 1 ½ tbsp grated parmesan cheese
- ¼ tsp salt
- 1/8 tsp ground black pepper
- 2 tsp avocado oil

Directions:

1. Turn on the oven, then set it to 375 degrees F and let it preheat.
2. Meanwhile, take a medium skillet pan, place it over medium heat, add oil and when hot, add sausage and cook for 5 minutes until cooked.

3. Meanwhile, crack the egg in a medium bowl, add salt, black pepper, and cheeses, reserving 1 tbsp cheddar cheese and whisk until mixed.

4. When the sausage has cooked, transfer it to the bowl containing egg batter and stir until combined.

5. Take a baking pan, grease it with oil, pour in sausage mixture, sprinkle remaining cheddar cheese in the top, and then bake for 10 to 12 minutes until cooked.

6. When done, let sausage cool for 5 minutes, then cut it into squares and then serve.

Nutrition: 439 Calories; 38.9 g Fats; 19.7 g Protein; 2.2 g Net Carb; 0 g Fiber;

41. Sausage and Marinara Casserole

Preparation time: 5 minutes

Cooking time: 12 minutes

Servings: 2

Ingredients:

- 2 oz chorizo
- 4 oz sausage
- 1 tbsp avocado oil
- 4 oz marinara sauce
- 2 tbsp grated cheddar cheese
- ¼ tsp salt
- 1/8 tsp ground black pepper
- ¼ tsp dried thyme

Directions:

1. Take a medium skillet pan, place it over medium heat, add oil and when hot, add chorizo and sausage and cook for 4 to 5 minutes until meat is no longer pink.
2. Add the marinara sauce into the pan, stir in salt, black pepper, and thyme, cook for 1 minute until

hot and then transfer meat mixture into a casserole dish.

3. Sprinkle cheese over the top of casserole and then bake for 7 minutes until thoroughly cooked.
4. Serve.

Nutrition: 485 Calories; 44.4 g Fats; 15.6 g Protein; 3.7 g Net Carb; 1.1 g Fiber;

POULTRY

42. Boozy Glazed Chicken

Preparation Time: 40 minutes

Cooking Time: 1 hour + marinating time

Servings: 4

Ingredients:

- 2 pounds chicken drumettes
- 2 tablespoons ghee, at room temperature
- Sea salt and ground black pepper, to taste
- 1 teaspoon Mediterranean seasoning mix
- 2 vine-ripened tomatoes, pureed
- 3/4 cup rum
- 3 tablespoons coconut aminos
- A few drops of liquid Stevia
- 1 teaspoon Chile peppers, minced
- 1 tablespoon minced fresh ginger
- 1 teaspoon ground cardamom
- 2 tablespoons fresh lemon juice, plus wedges for serving

Directions:

1. Toss the chicken with the melted ghee, salt, black pepper, and Mediterranean seasoning mix until well coated on all sides.
2. In another bowl, thoroughly combine the pureed tomato puree, rum, coconut aminos, Stevia, Chile peppers, ginger, cardamom, and lemon juice.
3. Pour the tomato mixture over the chicken drumettes; let it marinate for 2 hours. Bake in the preheated oven at 410 degrees F for about 45 minutes.
4. Add in the reserved marinade and place under the preheated broiler for 10 minutes.

Nutrition: 307 Calories 12.1g Fat 2.7g Carbs 33.6g Protein 1.5g Fiber

43. Festive Turkey Rouladen

Preparation Time: 15 minutes

Cooking Time: 30 minutes

Servings: 5

Ingredients:

- 2 pounds turkey fillet, marinated and cut into 10 pieces
- 10 strips prosciutto
- 1/2 teaspoon chili powder
- 1 teaspoon marjoram
- 1 sprig rosemary, finely chopped
- 2 tablespoons dry white wine
- 1 teaspoon garlic, finely minced
- 1 ½ tablespoons butter, room temperature
- 1 tablespoon Dijon mustard
- Sea salt and freshly ground black pepper, to your liking

Directions:

1. Start by preheating your oven to 430 degrees F.
2. Pat the turkey dry and cook in hot butter for about 3 minutes per side. Add in the mustard,

chili powder, marjoram, rosemary, wine, and garlic.

3. Continue to cook for 2 minutes more. Wrap each turkey piece into one prosciutto strip and secure with toothpicks.

4. Roast in the preheated oven for about 30 minutes.

Nutrition: 286 Calories 9.7g Fat 6.9g Carbs 39.9g Protein 0.3g Fiber

44. Pan-Fried Chorizo Sausage

Preparation Time: 10 minutes

Cooking Time: 20 minutes

Servings: 4

Ingredients:

- 16 ounces smoked turkey chorizo
- 1 ½ cups Asiago cheese, grated
- 1 teaspoon oregano
- 1 teaspoon basil
- 1 cup tomato puree
- 4 scallion stalks, chopped
- 1 teaspoon garlic paste
- Sea salt and ground black pepper, to taste
- 1 tablespoon dry sherry
- 1 tablespoon extra-virgin olive oil
- 2 tablespoons fresh coriander, roughly chopped

Directions:

1. Heat the oil in a frying pan over moderately high heat. Now, brown the turkey chorizo, crumbling with a fork for about 5 minutes.

2. Add in the other Ingredients, except for cheese; continue to cook for 10 minutes more or until cooked through.

Nutrition: 330 Calories 17.2g Fat 4.5g Carbs 34.4g Protein 1.6g Fiber

45. Chinese Bok Choy and Turkey Soup

Preparation Time: 15 minutes

Cooking Time: 40 minutes

Servings: 8

Ingredients:

- 1/2 pound baby Bok choy, sliced into quarters lengthwise
- 2 pounds turkey carcass
- 1 tablespoon olive oil
- 1/2 cup leeks, chopped
- 1 celery rib, chopped
- 2 carrots, sliced
- 6 cups turkey stock
- Himalayan salt and black pepper, to taste

Directions:

1. In a heavy-bottomed pot, heat the olive oil until sizzling. Once hot, sauté the celery, carrots, leek and Bok choy for about 6 minutes.
2. Add the salt, pepper, turkey, and stock; bring to a boil.

3. Turn the heat to simmer. Continue to cook, partially covered, for about 35 minutes.

Nutrition: 211 Calories 11.8g Fat 3.1g Carbs 23.7g Protein 0.9g Fiber

46. Herby Chicken Meatloaf

Preparation Time: 20 minutes

Cooking Time: 30 minutes

Servings: 6

Ingredients:

- 2 ½ lb. ground chicken
- 3 tbsp flaxseed meal
- 2 large eggs
- 2 tbsp olive oil
- 1 lemon,1 tbsp juiced
- ¼ cup chopped parsley
- ¼ cup chopped oregano
- 4 garlic cloves, minced
- Lemon slices to garnish

Directions:

1. Preheat oven to 400 F. In a bowl, combine ground chicken and flaxseed meal; set aside. In a small bowl, whisk the eggs with olive oil, lemon juice, parsley, oregano, and garlic.

2. Pour the mixture onto the chicken mixture and mix well. Spoon into a greased loaf pan and press to fit. Bake for 40 minutes.
3. Remove the pan, drain the liquid, and let cool a bit. Slice, garnish with lemon slices, and serve.

Nutrition: Cal 362 Net Carbs 1.3g Fat 24g Protein 35g

47. Lovely Pulled Chicken Egg Bites

Preparation Time: 15 minutes

Cooking Time: 30 minutes

Servings: 4

Ingredients:

- 2 tbsp butter
- 1 chicken breast
- 2 tbsp chopped green onions
- ½ tsp red chili flakes
- 12 eggs
- ¼ cup grated Monterey Jack

Directions:

1. Preheat oven to 400 F. Line a 12-hole muffin tin with cupcake liners. Melt butter in a skillet over medium heat and cook the chicken until brown on each side, 10 minutes.
2. Transfer to a plate and shred with 2 forks. Divide between muffin holes along with green onions and red chili flakes.

3. Crack an egg into each muffin hole and scatter the cheese on top. Bake for 15 minutes until eggs set. Serve.

Nutrition: Cal 393 Net Carbs 0.5g Fat 27g Protein 34g

48. Creamy Mustard Chicken with Shirataki

Preparation Time: 20 minutes

Cooking Time: 30 minutes

Servings: 4

Ingredients:

- 2 (8 oz.) packs angel hair shirataki
- 4 chicken breasts, cut into strips
- 1 cup chopped mustard greens
- 1 yellow bell pepper, sliced
- 1 tbsp olive oil
- 1 yellow onion, finely sliced
- 1 garlic clove, minced
- 1 tbsp wholegrain mustard
- 5 tbsp heavy cream
- 1 tbsp chopped parsley

Directions:

1. Boil 2 cups of water in a medium pot.
2. Strain the shirataki pasta and rinse well under hot running water. Allow proper draining and pour the shirataki pasta into the boiling water.

3. Cook for 3 minutes and strain again. Place a dry skillet and stir-fry the shirataki pasta until visibly dry, 1-2 minutes; set aside.
4. Heat olive oil in a skillet, season the chicken with salt and pepper and cook for 8-10 minutes; set aside. Stir in onion, bell pepper, and garlic and cook until softened, 5 minutes.
5. Mix in mustard and heavy cream; simmer for 2 minutes and mix in the chicken and mustard greens for 2 minutes. Stir in shirataki pasta, garnish with parsley and serve.

Nutrition: Cal 692 Net Carbs 15g Fats 38g Protein 65g

49. Parsnip & Bacon Chicken Bake

Preparation Time: 10 minutes

Cooking Time: 50 minutes

Servings: 4

Ingredients:

- 6 bacon slices, chopped
- 2 tbsp butter
- ½ lb. parsnips, diced
- 2 tbsp olive oil
- 1 lb. ground chicken
- 2 tbsp butter
- 1 cup heavy cream
- 2 oz. cream cheese, softened
- 1 ¼ cups grated Pepper Jack
- ¼ cup chopped scallions

Directions:

1. Preheat oven to 300 F. Put the bacon in a pot and fry it until brown and crispy, 6 minutes; set aside. Melt butter in a skillet and sauté parsnips until softened and lightly browned. Transfer to a greased baking sheet.

2. Heat olive oil in the same pan and cook the chicken until no longer pink, 8 minutes. Spoon onto a plate and set aside too.

3. Add heavy cream, cream cheese, and two-thirds of the Pepper Jack cheese to the pot. Melt the ingredients over medium heat, frequently stirring, 7 minutes.

4. Spread the parsnips on the baking dish, top with chicken, pour the heavy cream mixture over, and scatter bacon and scallions.

5. Sprinkle the remaining cheese on top and bake until the cheese melts and is golden, 30 minutes. Serve warm.

Nutrition: Cal 757 Net Carbs 5.5g Fat 66g Protein 29g

DESSERTS

50. Blackberry Cobbler

Preparation time: 5 minutes

Cooking time: 24 minutes

Servings: 6

Ingredients:

- 4 cups blackberries
- Juice of ½ lemon
- 2½ teaspoons liquid stevia, divided
- ¼ cup water
- 1 cup almond flour
- 4 tablespoons unsalted butter, melted
- ½ teaspoon cinnamon

Directions:

1. Place the blackberries, lemon juice, ½ teaspoon of liquid stevia, and water in the pot. Assemble the pressure lid, making sure the pressure release valve is in the SEAL position.

2. Select PRESSURE and set to HIGH. Set time to 5 minutes. Select START/STOP to begin.

3. While the berries are cooking, combine the almond flour, butter, cinnamon, and remaining 2 teaspoons of liquid stevia in a medium bowl. Using your hands, mix until moist.

4. When pressure cooking is complete, quick release the pressure by moving the pressure release valve to the VENT position. Carefully remove the lid when the unit has finished releasing pressure.

5. Sprinkle the crumble topping over the berry mixture.

6. Close the crisping lid. Select BROIL and set time to 10 minutes. Select START/STOP to begin, checking halfway through cooking to see how browning is progressing.

7. When cooking is complete, spoon the cobbler into bowls. Serve immediately.

Nutrition: Calories: 190; Total Fat: 14g; Total Carbohydrates: 12g; Fiber: 7g; Net Carbs: 5g; Protein: 4g; Erythritol Carbs: 2g Macronutrients: Fat: 66%; Protein: 9%; Carbs: 25%

51. Mocha Mousse

Preparation time: 2 hours and 35 minutes

Cooking time: 0

Servings: 4

Ingredients:

- For the Cream Cheese:
- Cream cheese, softened and full-fat – 8 ounces
- Sour cream, full-fat – 3 tablespoons
- Butter, softened – 2 tablespoons
- Vanilla extract, unsweetened – 1 ½ teaspoons
- Erythritol – 1/3 cup
- Cocoa powder, unsweetened – ¼ cup
- Instant coffee powder – 3 teaspoons
- For the Whipped Cream:
- Heavy whipping cream, full-fat – 2/3 cup
- Erythritol – 1 ½ teaspoon
- Vanilla extract, unsweetened – ½ teaspoon

Directions:

1. Prepare cream cheese mixture: For this, place cream cheese in a bowl, add sour cream and butter then beat until smooth.

2. Now add erythritol, cocoa powder, coffee, and vanilla and blend until incorporated, set aside until required.
3. Prepare whipping cream: For this, place whipping cream in a bowl and beat until soft peaks form.
4. Beat in vanilla and erythritol until stiff peaks form, then add 1/3 of the mixture into cream cheese mixture and fold until just mixed.
5. Then add remaining whipping cream mixture and fold until evenly incorporated.
6. Spoon the mousse into a freezer-proof bowl and place in the refrigerator for 2 ½ hours until set.
7. Serve straight away.

Nutrition: Calories: 421.7; Fat: 42 g; Protein: 6 g; Net Carbs: 6.5 g; Fiber: 2 g;

CPSIA information can be obtained
at www.ICGtesting.com
Printed in the USA
LVHW080146230521
688251LV00002B/195

9 781801 839884